MW00451720

Fighting Inflammatory Diseases
Inflammation Explained + Anti-Inflammatory Recipes

MELANIE FINLEY

Legal & Disclaimer

The information contained in this book and its contents is not designed to replace or take the place of any form of medical or professional advice; and is not meant to replace the need for independent medical, financial, legal or other professional advice or services, as may be required. The content and information in this book has been provided for educational and entertainment purposes only.

The content and information contained in this book has been compiled from sources deemed reliable, and it is accurate to the best of the Author's knowledge, information and belief. However, the Author cannot guarantee its accuracy and validity and cannot be held liable for any errors and/or omissions. Further, changes are periodically made to this book as and when needed. Where appropriate and/or necessary, you must consult a professional (including but not limited to your doctor, attorney, financial advisor or such other professional advisor) before using any of the suggested remedies, techniques, or information in this book.

Upon using the contents and information contained in this book, you agree to hold harmless the Author from and against any damages, costs, and expenses, including any legal fees potentially resulting from the application of any of the information provided by this book. This disclaimer applies to any loss, damages or injury caused by the use and application, whether directly or indirectly, of any advice or information presented, whether for breach of contract, tort, negligence, personal injury, criminal intent, or under any other cause of action.

You agree to accept all risks of using the information presented inside this book.

You agree that by continuing to read this book, where appropriate and/or necessary, you shall consult a professional (including but not limited to your doctor, attorney, or financial advisor or such other advisor as needed) before using any of the suggested remedies, techniques, or information in this book.

Table of Contents

Introduction..7

Types of inflammatory diseases..8

    Inflammatory diseases and oxidative stress..8

    Chronic inflammation and digestive system...8

    Inflammatory diseases and nutrition...8

    Inflammatory diseases and STD (sexually transmitted diseases)..............................9

    Inflammatory diseases and menopause 9

    Inflammatory diseases and environmental factors 9

What influences inflammatory diseases..10

The Anti Inflammatory Nutrient Chart 11

    Magnesium 11

    Beta Carotene and Vitamin A 12

    Quercetin 13

    Vitamin E 14

    Omega 3 Fats...14

    Vitamin D 15

    Vitamin C 15

    Zinc...16

Anti-inflammatory Food 18

    Bok Choy..19

    Celery 20

    Beets 20

    Broccoli 21

    Blueberries..22

    Pineapple 22

    Salmon..23

Bone broth 23

Walnuts 24

Coconut oil 24

Chia seeds 25

Flaxseeds 25

Turmeric 26

Ginger 26

Raw oats 27

Green tea 28

Dark chocolate 28

Red peppers 29

Black beans 30

Extra Virgin Olive Oil 31

Tomatoes 31

Whole grains 32

Eggs 32

Garlic 33

Oysters 33

Yogurt 34

Apples 34

Raw honey 35

Miso 36

Anti-inflammatory Diet **37**

High Protein food 38

Low Carbohydrates Food 39

Anti-inflammatory Recipes **40**

Anti-inflammatory Meals 41

Turmeric Chicken and Quinoa 41

Buddha Bowl 43

Cannellini beans with garlic and sage 45

Lemon basil baked garlic butter salmon 46

Blueberry Salmon Salad 48

Turmeric falafel 50

Green edamame spinach hummus pesto 52

Deep dish falafel pizza 54

Crunchy fresh broccoli quinoa salad 56

Kale and chickpea stuffed spaghetti squash 58

Beet and Quinoa Burgers 60

Sweet potato "rice" in Deep Dish 62

Golden roasted cauliflower and chickpeas 64

Curried tofu 65

Anti-inflammatory Snacks 68

Coconut and sweet potato muffins with cinnamon, ginger and maple syrup 68

Golden milk chia pudding 69

Golden turmeric milk chia seed pudding 71

Paleo ginger spiced muffins 73

Winter fruit salad 75

Coconut turmeric bites 76

Strawberry chia seed jam 78

Smooth chocolate chia pudding 80

Pomegranate ginger gummies 81

Baked zucchini chips 82

Anti-inflammatory Smoothies 85

    Cherry Mango Smoothie 85

    Green smoothie...86

    Pineapple ginger turmeric smoothie 87

    Turmeric golden milk smoothie 89

    Kiwi smoothie 91

    Frozen cranberry orange smoothie 93

Conclusion **95**

Check Out Other Books **96**

Introduction

Inflammation is the way that your body reacts to protect itself from harmful stimuli, including irritants, damaged cells or pathogens. Infection is different from inflammation. Infections occur when virus, bacteria or fungi invade your body, whereas inflammation occurs when your body fights to remove those invaders.

There are also certain foods that we eat, and which develop and lead to inflammatory diseases, such as red meat, high fat dairy products and fat (saturated and trans).

One of the most potent inflammatory sources can be the food we eat. First of all we can do a great deal to help reduce inflammation by eating more anti-inflammatory foods.

Everyone's choices about the food they eat have a great effect on their health. It's true that harmful foods tastes great but let's take a second and think about consequences over our health.

This e-book is created to guide you towards healthy food that has an effective way of diminishing and managing inflammation. It contains full color photography and complete nutritional information.

We are writing this e-book because people are confronting more and more with inflammatory diseases and they should know what they can eat to reduce inflammatory diseases.

"You are what you eat"

Types of inflammatory diseases

Even if the list of inflammatory diseases is long, certain conditions are more common.

Inflammatory diseases and oxidative stress

Inflammation is the result of an oxidative stress that aggresses cells and prevents them from functioning normally. In general, oxidative stress is the basis of many diseases, not just the basis of inflammatory diseases, which is why in recent years there has been an increasing awareness of antioxidants (substances that create a protective barrier against oxidative stress).

Inflammation may have such complex effects that sometimes it is difficult to establish a circuit of disease causes. For example, the incidence of arthero-sclerosis, myocardial infarction and stroke is increased at people suffering from rheumatoid arthritis, a condition caused by oxidative stress.

Chronic inflammation and digestive system

Surprisingly or not, the digestive system functions as a central know in its relationship with the rest of the body. If something does not work properly in the digestive system, the effects will not only be seen there, but also in other areas of the body. It's like a domino game. Two-thirds of the body's immune system is sustained by the way the gastrointestinal tract works, and yet the digestive system is often the last place where the cause of the inflammatory disease is sought.

Gastrointestinal disorders, diarrhea, constipation, bloating, flatulence, abdominal pain, stomach burning and gastroesophageal reflux are some of the first signs of digestive tract inflammation.

No wonder the digestive system controls much of the body's resistance, since its function is to eliminate viruses, bacteria, toxins and other harmful substances before they affect the entire body. Inflammatory bowel disease (Chron disease, ulcero-hemorrhagic-rectocolitis) occurs when the digestive system clogs under the burden of factors that aggravate bad habits, eating, sedentariness etc.

Inflammatory diseases and nutrition

Food is the most important factor that leads to inflammation, but not all food products have negative effects. Food additives, fast food, red meat, white sugar, white flour, white pasta, white rice and many other foods that undergo a refining process are a certain point causing the development of inflammatory diseases in vulnerable body areas.

Many of the polyunsaturated vegetable oils, such as sunflower oil, peanut oil, corn oil and soybean oil, contain a high amount of linoleic acid, an essential omega-6 fatty acid, which the body turns it into Arachidonic acid, which favors inflammation.

By comparison, essential omega-3 fatty acids are known for their anti-inflammatory effects. Our ancestors had a diet of omega-6 and omega-3 in the ratio of 11. Currently, the proportion of essential fatty acids in the diet of the majority of the population is between 101 and 251.

For most people, eating high in carbohydrates and low in protein is one that causes the development of inflammatory diseases.

Refined sugar and other foods with high glycemic levels quickly increase insulin levels and put the immune system in the alert, making it vulnerable to risk factors.

Inflammatory diseases and STD (sexually transmitted diseases)

Sexually transmitted diseases may also be blamed for the occurrence of inflammatory diseases.

For example, STDs can cause inflammation or infection of upper reproductive organs in women, i.e. pelvic inflammatory disease. Bacterial vaginosis is also a cause that can cause pelvic inflammatory disease.

Inflammatory diseases and menopause

Aging at women favors the emergence of inflammatory diseases. Around the menopause, the risk of osteoporosis is higher because of changes occurring at the hormonal level.

Estrogen, progesterone and testosterone have varying levels, which can lead to apathy and inflammation of the bone system.

Inflammatory diseases and environmental factors

Sometimes, the environment has also a negative role on the body and can lead to the development of inflammatory diseases. It is enough for a person to enter a space with a chemical smell and a headache is installed. Basically, headache is nothing but an inflammation, which is temporary.

Pollution, synthetic materials, adhesives, plastic, room fresheners, house-hold cleaners, pesticides are substances that the world is hit by every day. Little by little, they begin to aggress the body and produce that oxidative stress so harmful to each person.

What influences inflammatory diseases

1. Low level of glutathione (the peptide that contains amino acids and plays an important role in the oxido-reduction reaction)

2. Low levels of vitamin D and antioxidant substances

3. Increased levels of oxidized glutathione

4. A high level of malondialdehyde (a marker of oxidative stress that is formed when fats are oxidized)

5. Increased lipid peroxidation

6. High level of homocysteine

7. High levels of fructosamine

8. Isoprostane (markers of oxidative stress that are formed when fats are oxidized)

The listed scientific terms may sound confusing or hard to understand. But in conclusion, these are the after effects of the unhealthy food you consumed daily.

The Anti Inflammatory Nutrient Chart

Based on researches done from the medical websites, here are some important facts on various vitamin and minerals that are found in your daily consumed food; the lowest figure means most anti-inflammatory.

Food / Vitamin / Mineral	Inflammatory Weightage
Magnesium	-0.905
Turmeric	-0.774
Beta Carotene	-0.725
Vitamin A	-0.58
Tea	-0.552
Fibre	-0.52
Quercetin	-0.49
Wine	-0.49
Vitamin E	-0.401
Omega 3 fats	-0.384
Vitamin C	-0.342
Vitamin D	-0.367
Zinc	-0.316
Vitamin B6	-0.286
Garlic	-0.27
Ginger	-0.18
Riboflavin	-0.16
Protein	-0.5
Caffeine	-0.35
Iron	-0.29

Let's drill into more detail for few main items listed above.

Magnesium

Being the highest in the rank of anti-inflammatory nutrient, let's take a look at the food that contains the high magnesium level.

Vegetables	Amount (mg)
Seaweed	218
Potatoes	196
Spinach	157
Tomatoes	105
Kale	74

Sweet potato	61
Pumpkin	56
Beetroot	39
Fruits	**Amount (mg)**
Tamarinds	110
Bananas	108
Figs	101
Prunes	84
Grapefruit	79
Avocadoes	67
Gluten free grains	**Amount (mg)**
Brown rice	177
Millet flour	142
Quinoa	118
Brown rice	86
Wild rice	52
Beans and legumes	**Amount (mg)**
Chickpea	153
Tempeh	134
Lima beans	126
Navy beans	105
Pinto beans	56

Beta Carotene and Vitamin A

Beta Carotene is a version of Vitamin A. Here is a list of food with high contents in Beta carotene and Vitamin A.

Food	Amount (mg per cup)
Sweet potato –peeled	31.0
Sweet potato baked in skin	25.1
Peas and carrots frozen	13.1
Carrots, kale – boiled	12.0
Spinach – boiled	11.2
Kale – boiled	10.5
Raw carrots	10.6
Mustard greens	10.4
Butternut Squash/pumpkin baked	9.4
Collards- boiled	8.6
Beet Greens	6.6

Turnip greens	6.6
Chinese cabbage	4.3

Quercetin

Quercetin is a flavonoid. A flavonoid is a group of plant pigments that give fruits and vegetables their color. Flavonoids are powerful antioxidants that help the body fight free radicals, which can damage cells.

Here is a list of food with high contents of Quercetin.

Food	Amount (mg per cup)
Dill	55.16
Buckwheat	23.09
Cacao powder	20.13
Red onions	19.36
Spring onions	14.24
Cranberries (raw)	14.02
Tarragon	10.0
Kale (raw)	7.71
White onion	5.19
Coriander (raw)	5.0
Spinach (raw)	4.86
Chives (raw)	4.77
Apples	4.42
Tomato puree	4.12
Watercress (raw)	4.0
Red grapes	3.54
Celery	3.50
Broccoli – raw	3.21
Blueberries	3.11
Cherry tomatoes	2.77
Green beans (raw)	2.73
Buckwheat flour – Wholegrain	2.72
Green tea	2.69
Apricot	2.55
Black grapes	2.54
Iceberg lettuce	2.47
Lemons	2.29
Loose-leaf lettuce	1.95
Cherries	1.25
Plums	1.20
Broccoli – cooked	1.0

Vitamin E

This is both an antioxidant and anti-inflammatory. It's most helpful for chronic skin conditions, especially with vitamins C and D.

Food	Amount (mg per cup)
Seaweed – spirulina	5.60
Tomato puree	4.92
Frozen spinach	4.70
Taro	4.03
Spinach	3.74
Tomatoes	3.74
Turnip greens	3.47
Lambs quarter	3.36
Chard	3.31
Red bell pepper	3.22
Sweet potato – boiled	3.08
Canned asparagus drained	2.95
Butternut squash	2.64
Mustard greens	2.49
Broccoli	2.48

Omega 3 Fats

It is commonly known that omega-3 fatty acids are good for the brain. However, omega 3 contains two contents - eicosapentaenoic acid (EPA) and docosahexaenoic acid (DHA) which serves an important role in reduction of cellular inflammation.

Here is a list of food that has high content in EPA & DHA.

Food	Amount (EPA – g)	Amount (DHA)
Mackerel	2.202	4.032
Herring	1.788	1.272
Red salmon fillets - with skin	0.977	1.642
Sablefish	0.737	0.792
Pink salmon - canned	0.718	0.685

Tinned sardines	0.705	0.758
Halibut fish	0.573	0.429
Tuna - canned	0.198	0.880
Cold pressed flaxseed oil	53.38g Alpha Linoleic Acid	

Vitamin D

Vitamin D can be easily obtained from the sunlight. But due to the climate change caused by global warming, we try to avoid going into direct sunlight to protect ourselves from UV light. Applying sunblock will also mean blocking the absorption of vitamin D.

Not many people know that adequate cholesterol is required for efficient conversion of vitamin D, and this is highly unlikely to be accepted by most people.

Therefore, maximizing intake of vitamin D rich foods became vital to most people. Here is a list of food source that contain high contents for vitamin D.

Note: IU refers to "International Unit". Click HERE to understand more.

Food	Amount (IU per cup)
Mackerel	1368
Halibut	1360
Maitake Mushrooms	786
Red salmon tinned	715
Portabella mushrooms	539
Trout	539
Canned pink salmon –drained	493
Catfish	425
Canned tuna in olive oil – drained	393
Canned sardines	288
Eggs	118

Vitamin C

Vitamin C is a powerful antioxidant that helps boost the body's immune system, prevent damage to our bodies from toxicities and pollutants. It is necessary for proper growth and to heal wounds. It creates collagen tissue for healthy gums, teeth, bones and blood vessels.

Here is a list if food with high Vitamin C content.

Vegetables	Amount (mg)
Yellow peppers	341.3
Red peppers	230.8
Green peppers	217.6
Mustard spinach	195
Broccoli	106.2
Kohlrabi	89.0
Kale	87.1
Fruits	Amount (mg)
Guava	376.7
Kiwifruit	166.9
Litchis	135.8
Lemons	112.4
Oranges	97.5
Pineapple	93.1
Strawberries	89.4
Papaya	88.3
Grapefruit	85.1

Zinc

Zinc is both an antioxidant and anti-Inflammatory agent to human health.

Zinc supplementation works to decrease oxidative stress biomarkers and inflammatory cytokines especially for the elderly.

Here is a list of food with high zinc contents.

Food	Amount (mg per 100g)
Mollusks, oysters (eastern)	90.95
Mollusks, oysters (pacific)	16.62
Beef	12.28
Veal	12.00
Sesame seed paste – unroasted	10.45
Pumpkin seeds	10.30
Sesame seeds	10.23

Always take care of your health. If you're busy and unable to prepare food at home, you should use the following calculator to check on the nutrition facts before you decide whether to go ahead to order the food. This is easy to use but you will need Internet access.

https://www.nutritionvalue.org/nutritioncalculator.php

Otherwise, you may search and download nutrition calculator Apps either from Android or Apple store.

Anti-inflammatory Food

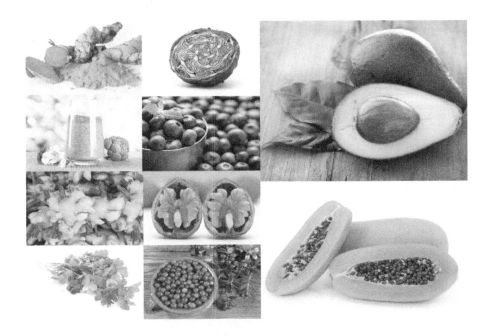

Clinical studies have shown that some foods may be beneficial in reducing inflammation.

Foods considered anti-inflammatory contain nutrients that fight effectively against physical pain – head, bones, back, joint – caused by internal inflammation that can appear in the body. Nutritionists claim that these foods should be part of every person's diet, not just for this benefit, but for many other therapeutic properties they have for the body.

Some of the food listed below includes the nutrient contents for your reference.

Note: DV refers to the "Daily Value" – which is the amount required of an average person for each day.

Green leafy vegetables

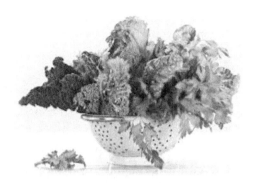

These operate as anti-inflammatory flavonoids and are rich in antioxidants that restore cellular health.

Anti-Inflammatory content (DV per cup)	
Vitamin K	639%
Vitamin A	60%
Vitamin C	42%

Bok Choy

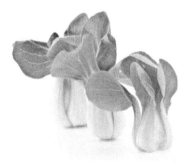

t's an excellent source of antioxidant vitamins, minerals and antioxidants. Studies show over 70 antioxidant phenolic substances in bok choy.

Anti-Inflammatory content (DV per cup)	
Vitamin K	64%
Vitamin A	59%
Vitamin C	40%

Celery

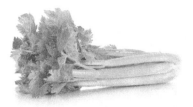

Celery demonstrates both antioxidant and anti-inflammatory activities that help improve blood pressure and cholesterol levels. Celery seeds help lower inflammation and fight bacterial infections.

Anti-Inflammatory content (DV per cup)	
Vitamin K	37%
Vitamin A	9%
Vitamin C	5%
Potassium	8%

Beets

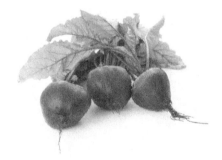

The antioxidant Betalain gives beets their color and they are an excellent anti-inflammatory. Their inflammatory compounds inhibit the activity of cyclooxygenase enzymes.

Anti-Inflammatory content (DV per cup)	
Folate	34%
Manganese	28%
Potassium	15%
Magnesium	10%

Broccoli

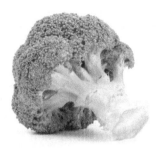

Broccoli is an antioxidant powerhouse. It works together with its 2 key vitamins, carotenoids and flavonoids to lower oxidative stress in the body.

Anti-Inflammatory content (DV per cup)	
Vitamin K	254%
Vitamin C	135%
Chromium	53%
Folate	42%
Vitamin B6	18%
Vitamin E	15%
Manganese	15%
Vitamin A	13%

Blueberries

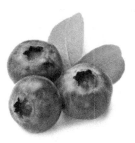

Blueberries contain quercetin, a flavonoid that fights inflammation and even cancer. Studies show that consuming blueberries slowed cognitive decline and improved memory and motor function.

Anti-Inflammatory content (DV per cup)	
Vitamin K	64%
Vitamin A	59%
Vitamin C	40%

Pineapple

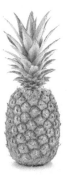

Pineapples contain bromelain – a digestive enzyme – which is observed to have immune-modulating abilities. Bromelain stops blood platelets from sticking together or building up along the walls of blood vessels.

Anti-Inflammatory content (DV per cup)	
Vitamin C	131%
Manganese	79%

Salmon

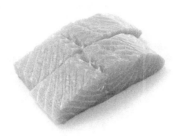

Salmon is a great source of essential fatty acids, especially omega-3, which are some of the most potent anti-inflammatory substances.

Omega-3 fatty acids reduce inflammation and may help lower risk of chronic diseases.

Anti-Inflammatory content (DV per four-serving)	
Vitamin B12	236%
Vitamin D	127%
Selenium	78.3%
Vitamin B3	56.3%
Omega-3	55%
Protein	53.1%
Phosphorus	52.1%
Vitamin B6	37.6%

Bone broth

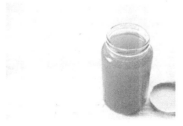

Bone broths contain minerals in forms that your body can absorb easily. They contain chondroitin sulphates and glucosamine, compounds that reduce inflammation.

Walnuts

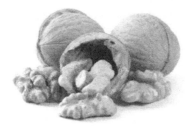

The antioxidant and anti-inflammatory benefits of walnuts help protect you against metabolic syndrome, cardiovascular problems and Type-2 diabetes.

Anti-Inflammatory content (DV per cup)	
Omega-3	452%
Manganese	204%

Coconut oil

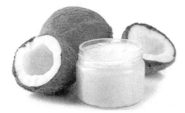

Lipids from the coconut oil are full of strong anti-inflammatory compounds. It contains 95% unsaturated fats.

Chia seeds

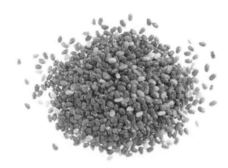

Chia seeds offer both omega-3 and omega-6, which should be consumed in balance with one another. They are beneficial to consumption because their ability to reverse inflammation, regulate cholesterol and lower blood pressure.

Anti-Inflammatory content (DV for every 3 tbsp)	
Omega-3	883%
Omega-6	710%

Flaxseeds

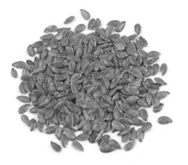

Beside the fact that being an excellent source of omega-3 and phytonutrients, flaxseeds are also packed with antioxidants.

Anti-Inflammatory content (DV for every 3 tbsp)	
Omega-3	1168%
Vitamin B1	31%
Manganese	35%
Magnesium	30%
Phosphorus	19%

Turmeric

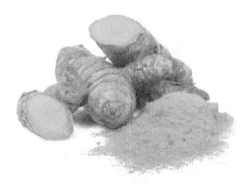

The active anti-inflammatory component from turmeric si curcumin, a component that is far more potent than aspirin and ibuprofen

Anti-Inflammatory content (DV for every 2 tsp)	
Manganese	17%
Vitamin B6	5%

Ginger

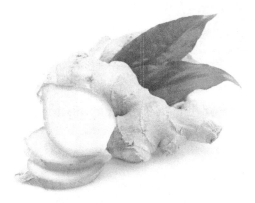

Ginger can be used fresh, dried or in supplement form and extracts.

Ginger is an immune modulator that helps reduce inflammation caused by overactive immune responses.

Ginger has the ability to break down the accumulation of toxins in your organs.

Anti-Inflammatory content (DV per 100g)	
Protein	4%
Vitamin C	8%
Iron	3%
Magnesium	11%
Manganese	11%
Potassium	9%
Zinc	2%

Raw oats

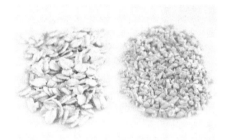

Raw oats are a resistant starch, a type of carbohydrate that passes through your gut undigested. It feeds your healthy gut bacteria, which in turn produce a fatty acid that encourages more efficient fat oxidation known as butyrate. Higher levels of butyrate reduce inflammation in your body and help reduce insulin resistance as well.

Anti-Inflammatory content (DV per 100g)	
Protein	34%
Iron	30%
Vitamin B6	8%
Magnesium	59%
Manganese	282%
Phosphorus	73%
Potassium	12%
Zinc	21%

Green tea

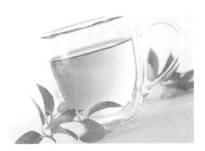

Scientific studies suggest that the high EGCG (epigallocatechin gallate) and polyphenol content in green tea make it a stronger anti-inflammatory elixir than other teas like black tea.

These anti-inflammatory properties have also been implicated in preventing the development and growth of skin tumors.

Anti-Inflammatory content (DV per cup)	
Manganese	23%
Magnesium	1%
Protein	1%
Magnesium	1%
Vitamin B6	1%

Dark chocolate

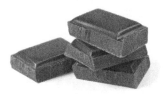

Cocoa contains antioxidants that prevents weight gain and lower the blood sugar levels.

In a study at Louisiana State University, it was found that the gut microbes in our stomach ferment chocolate into compounds that are heart-healthy and anti-inflammatory. The compounds actually shut down genes that are linked to insulin resistance and inflammation.

Anti-Inflammatory content (DV per 100g)	
Protein	16%
Iron	66%
Vitamin B12	5%

Vitamin K	9%
Iron	66%
Magnesium	57%
Manganese	97%
Phosphorus	31%
Potassium	15%

Red peppers

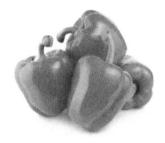

Red peppers contain high amount of inflammatory-biomarker - reducing vitamin C along with the bioflavonoids beta-carotene, quercetin and luteolin.

Luteolin helps to neutralize free radicals and reduce inflammation.

Anti-Inflammatory content (DV per 100g)	
Protein	2%
Vitamin C	213%
Magnesium	3%
Manganese	6%
Phosphorus	3%
Potassium	4%
Vitamin B6	15%
Vitamin A	63%

Black beans

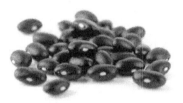

Black beans provide the energy source for your healthy bugs to ferment into the inflammation-reducing fatty acid butyrate.

They are high in anthocyanins, antioxidants which have also been associated with lowering inflammation.

Anti-Inflammatory content (DV per 100g)	
Protein	6%
Vitamin C	13%
Iron	5%
Phosphorus	8%
Potassium	4%
Zinc	4%

Extra Virgin Olive Oil

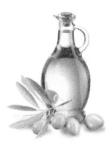

Oleocanthal is found only in extra virgin olive oil and has a significant impact on inflammation and helps reduce joint cartilage damage, working similarly to ibuprofen.

Tomatoes

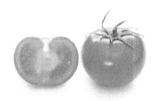

Tomatoes contain lycopene, an antioxidant that protects your brain and fights depression-causing inflammation.

Anti-Inflammatory content (DV per Tomato 111g)	
Vitamin A	33%
Vitamin C	30%
Protein	3%
Iron	3%
Magnesium	2%
Manganese	3%
Phosphorus	3%
Potassium	3%

Whole grains

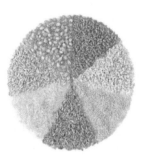

Brown rice, quinoa, millet and amaranth, all are packed with fiber that helps produce butyrate, a fatty acid that runs off genes related to inflammation and insulin resistance. The high B vitamin content of whole grains also helps to reduce the inflammatory hormone homocysteine in the body.

Eggs

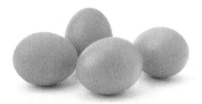

Vitamin D from the eggs fends off depression and cold, reduces the risk of certain cancers and diminishes inflammation.

The yolk contains a host of fat-blasting and health-boosting nutrients from vitamin D to fat-blasting choline.

Anti-Inflammatory content (DV per large egg)	
Protein	13%
Iron	5%
Vitamin A	6%
Vitamin B12	8%
Vitamin B6	4%
Vitamin D	10%
Phosphorus	10%
Zinc	5%

Garlic

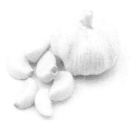

Garlic helps to stimulate anti-inflammatory proteins that suppress the inflammatory markers in chronic inflammation environments.

Anti-Inflammatory content (DV per clove)	
Vitamin B6	2%
Vitamin C	2%
Manganese	2%

Oysters

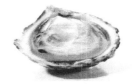

SOD (superoxide dismutase enzyme) works as an antioxidant to deactivating free-radicals and cell-damaging. To function properly, it works hand in hand with three minerals: zinc, copper, manganese.

Oysters are also a great source of omega-3.

Anti-Inflammatory content (DV per 100g)	
Protein	46%
Iron	31%
Phosphorus	22%
Zinc	40%
Vitamin B12	113%
Vitamin B6	32%

Yogurt

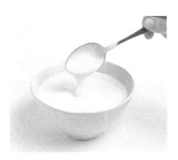

Adding cultured, fermented foods into your diet can recolonize your gut with beneficial microbes, which can assist with fending off inflammation.

Low sugar yogurt is one of the most accessible sources of probiotics, but you can also consume kefir, sauerkraut pickles, kimchi and cheese.

Anti-Inflammatory content (DV per cup)	
Protein	34%
Vitamin B12	21%
Vitamin B6	5%
Magnesium	5%
Phosphorus	23%
Zinc	6%

Apples

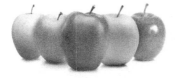

Apple peels are full of pectin, a natural fruit fiber that is found to be powerful enough to support the growth of the beneficial bacteria.

Also, apple peels provide an average of 10mg of quercetin boosting, anti-inflammatory oxidant.

Anti-Inflammatory content (DV per large apple)	
Vitamin C	17%
Vitamin A	2%

Iron	2%
Magnesium	3%
Manganese	4%
Phosphorus	2%
Potassium	5%
Zinc	1%

Raw honey

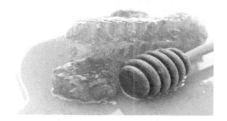

Honey contains proteolytic enzymes that are essential when it comes to modulating the inflammatory response.

Honey is one of the best sources of these enzymes because it is made by bee's enzyme-rich saliva.

It is also full of anti-inflammatory carotenoids, polyphenols, vitamins and antioxidants.

Anti-Inflammatory content (DV per tbsp)	
Protein	2%
Vitamin C	3%
Iron	8%
Manganese	14%
Potassium	4%
Zinc	5%

Miso

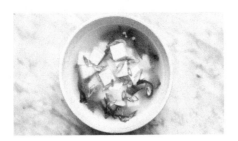

Not only that miso is a fermented food which means it is rich in probiotic compounds, but it's also made from soy.

Studies suggested that soy's isoflavones may be powerful anti-inflammatories.

Anti-Inflammatory content (DV per 100g)	
Protein	15%
Iron	7%
Vitamin B6	29%
Magnesium	15%
Manganese	33%
Phosphorus	21%
Potassium	15%
Zinc	7%

Anti-inflammatory Diet

YES FOODS	NO FOODS
Vegetables: Raw, Steamed, Sautéed, Juiced, Baked vegetables	Canned or creamed in casseroles / deep dish
Fats: Flax seeds oil, Olive oil , Cold/expeller – pressed canola, Sesame, Sunflower, Safflower, Almond oil, Walnut, Pumpkin, Dressings made from these oils	Butter, margarine, shortening, , salad dressing, processed oil, spreads
Beverages: 8 cups of filtered/distilled water/day, Herbal tea	Coffee, tea, Soda pop, alcoholic beverages, all caffeinated beverages
Spices: Cinnamon, Parsley, Cumin, Dill, Garlic, Ginger, Oregano, Thyme, Rosemary, Tarragon, Turmeric	Cayenne pepper, paprika
Sweeteners: Brown rice syrup, Fruit sweetener, Molasses	No white/brown refined sugar, honey, corn syrup, maple syrup, high fructose corn syrup
Fruits: unsweetened fresh, frozen or water-packed, canned fruits, fruit juices	All citrus fruits: grapes, oranges, lemon, grapefruit and lime, fruit drinks, dried fruits
Starch: non-gluten grain (brown rice, millet, quinoa, amaranth, tapioca, buckwheat)	Spelt, wheat, barely, corn, oats, kamut, rye and all gluten-containing products
Bread/ cereal: any made from rice, buckwheat, millet, soy, tapioca, arrowroot, amaranth, quinoa	All wheat, oat, spelt, kamut, rye, barely, or gluten containing products
Meat: all fresh fish such as halibut, salmon, cod, sole, trout; wild game, chicken, turkey, lamb	Beef, pork, cold cuts, frankfurters, sausage, canned meats, eggs, shellfish
Nuts and seeds: almonds, cashews, walnut, sesame, sunflower, pumpkin, nut butters made from these seeds	Peanuts, pistachios, peanut butter
Dairy products: milk substitutes such as rice milk, soy milk, nut milk	Milk, cheese, cottage cheese, cream,, butter, ice cream, non-dairy creamer.

High Protein food

MEAT	FISH	DAIRY
Bison	Trout	Almond milk
Eggs	Sardines	Unsweetened
Chicken	Cod	Coconut milk
Duck	Salmon	Organic cow milk
Lamb	Tilapia	Organic cow cheese
Turkey	Haddock	Organic Greek
Venison	Halibut	yogurt
Elk	Tuna	Goat milk
Veal	Grouper	Goat cheese
	Sea bass	Goat yogurt
	Mackerel	Kefir
	Mahi-mahi	Sheep cheese
	Red snapper	Sheep yogurt
	Walleye	

Low Carbohydrates Food

VEGETABLES		FRUITS
Artichoke	Kale	All berries
Arugula	Mushrooms	Apple
Asparagus	Mustard greens	Orange
Beets	Onions	Pears
Bell peppers	Okra	Lemon
Bok choy	Romaine lettuce	Lime
Broccoli	Parsnip	
Brussels sprouts	Peas	
Cabbage	Peppers	
Carrots	Pumpkin	
Celery	Radish	
Collards	Spinach	
Cucumber	Squash	
Eggplant	Tomatoes	
Garlic	Turnip greens	
Green beans	Watercress	

Anti-inflammatory Recipes

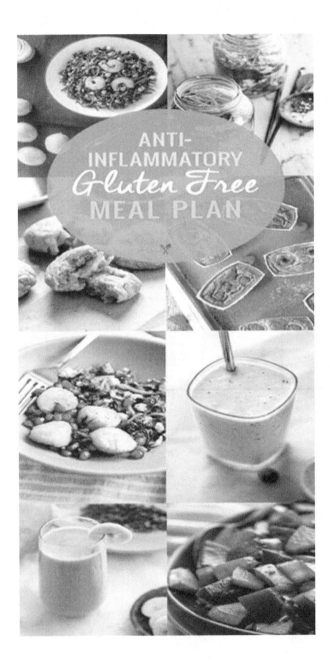

Following a diet that's full of anti-inflammatory foods can help you control and alleviate some of you inflammatory diseases. Bring on your attention to these recipes and let's get started. Take note that the "%" presented in nutrition facts are "Percent Daily Values" which are based on a 2000 calorie diet.

Anti-inflammatory Meals

Turmeric Chicken and Quinoa

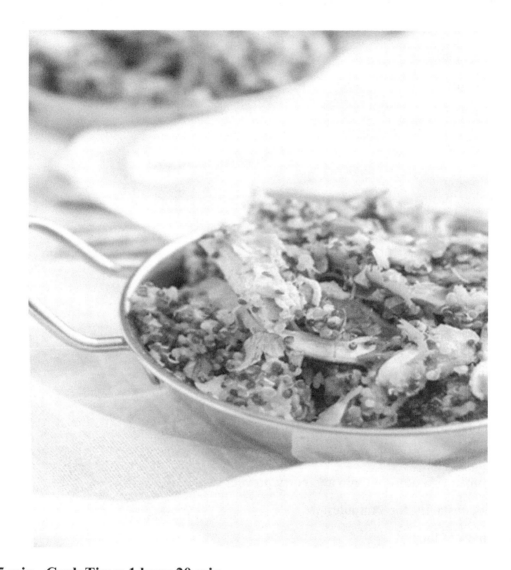

Prep Time: 25 min   Cook Time: 1 hour 20 min

Servings: 6

Ingredients:

- 2 pounds skinless boneless chicken
- 1 tsp salt
- ½ tsp fresh ground black pepper

- 1 tsp ground turmeric
- 1 chopped onion
- 1 tbsp extra virgin oil
- 1 tbsp grated fresh peeled chopped ginger
- 2 plum chopped tomatoes
- 4 cloves minced garlic
- ½ tsp ground cumin
- 1 ½ tsp curry powder
- 2 cups rinsed quinoa
- 2 bay leaves
- 2 ¾ cups chicken broth
- 1 ½ tbsp Asian fish sauce

Instructions:

1. Season the chicken with salt and pepper
2. In a large oven, heat olive oil to medium. Add turmeric and stir
3. Put in the chicken
4. Cook until brown on both sides
5. Transfer to a plate and allow to cool. Shred it
6. Add ginger and onion. Cook for 8 minutes
7. Add garlic, tomatoes, quinoa, cumin and curry powder
8. Cook and stir constantly for 3 minutes
9. Put chicken back to the pot
10. Add fish sauce, bay leaves, and chicken broth
11. Bring to a simmer
12. Cover and cook over low heat for 25 minutes
13. Remove let stand covered for 5 minutes
14. Serve it!
15. Cheers!

Nutrition Facts (Per serving):

• Calories	455
• Sodium	3733mg
• Fat	8.1g
• Potassium	484mg
• Carbohydrate	44.9g
• Fiber	5.2g
• Sugars	6g
• Protein	48.6g
• Cholesterol	95mg
• Calcium	44mg
• Iron	3mg

Buddha Bowl

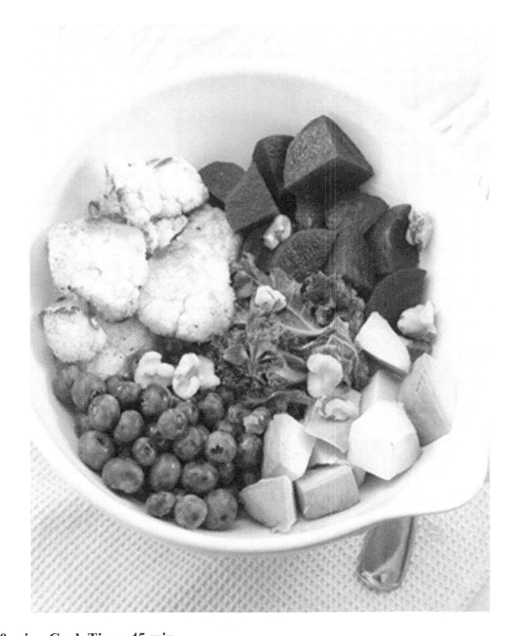

Prep Time: 20 min   Cook Time: 45 min

Servings: 4

Ingredients:

- 2 1/2 lb. cauliflower - cut into chunks
- 2 avocados

- 2c blueberries
- $1/3$ cup chopped raw walnuts
- 7 medium cooked beets - peeled and quartered
- 1 tbsp extra virgin olive oil
- 10 oz. chopped kale
- 1 tsp turmeric
- Salt and pepper
- 1 clove garlic

Instructions:

1. Preheat oven to 425F
2. Cover a baking sheet with foil. Spray with olive oil. Set aside
3. In a large bowl, add cauliflower and olive oil. Stir well
4. Sprinkle in turmeric and mix
5. Spread cauliflower over baking sheet
6. Sprinkle generously with sea salt and pepper as well as a little cayenne pepper and nutritional yeast
7. Bake cauliflower for about 30 minutes
8. Slightly before 30 minutes, heat a large fry pan with a small drizzle of oil or a little coconut oil spray over medium heat
9. Add in kale. Toss until wilt and grate in garlic
10. Toss to coat
11. Cut avocado into chunks
12. Portion kale among bowls
13. Top with blueberries, roasted turmeric cauliflower, avocado, beets and walnuts
14. Serve it!
15. Cheers!

Nutrition Facts (Per serving):

•	**Calories**	508
•	**Sodium**	236mg

•	Fat	30.1g
•	Potassium	2133mg
•	Carbohydrate	56.8g
•	Fiber	19.2g
•	Sugars	26.8g
•	Protein	14.3g
•	Cholesterol	0mg
•	Calcium	191mg
•	Iron	6mg

Cannellini beans with garlic and sage

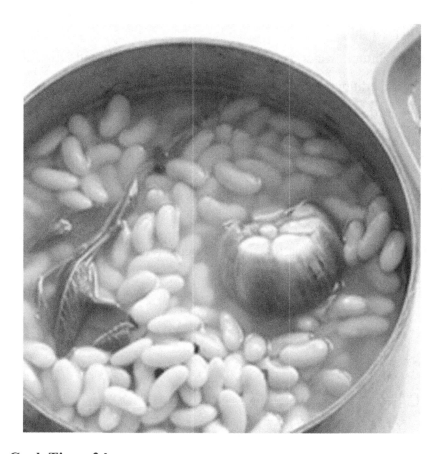

Prep Time: 20 min   Cook Time: 3 hours

Servings: 6

Ingredients:

- 1 lb. dried, white kidney beans
- 1 large fresh sage sprig
- 1 large head of garlic, unpeeled - cut off the top to expose cloves
- ¼ tsp whole black peppercorns
- 8 cups room-temperature water
- 2 tbsp olive oil
- Extra virgin oil (for drizzling)
- 1 tsp coarse kosher salt

Instructions:

1. Soak beans in large bowl with cold water – leaves over night
2. Drain the water and pour into a large pot
3. Add 8 cups room-temperature water, garlic, sage, black peppercorns and 2tbsp olive oil
4. Bring to simmer over medium heat.
5. Reduce heat to medium-low
6. Simmer uncovered for 30 minutes, stir occasionally
7. Add in 1 tsp coarse salt
8. Continue to simmer until beans are tender. Keep beans covered for another 30 minutes.
9. Cool beans in liquid for 1 hour
10. Transfer beans to bowl, discarding garlic, sage and peppercorns. Season beans to taste with pepper and more coarse salt. Drizzle with extra virgin oil
11. Serve it!
12. Cheers!

Nutrition Facts (Per serving):

• **Calories**	218
• **Sodium**	86mg
• **Fat**	7.6g
• **Potassium**	635mg
• **Carbohydrate**	28.8g
• **Fiber**	7.3g
• **Sugars**	1g
• **Protein**	10.5g
• **Cholesterol**	0mg
• **Calcium**	51mg
• **Iron**	3mg

Lemon basil baked garlic butter salmon

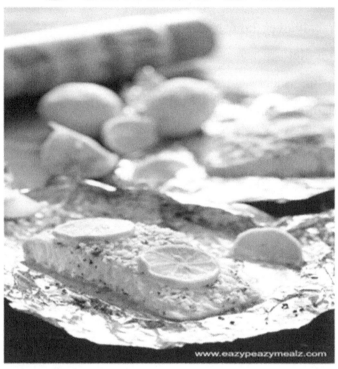

Prep Time: 10 min   Cook Time: 45 min

Serving: 3 (2 pieces of salmon per serving)

Ingredients:

- 6 pieces of salmon
- 2 lemons
- ½ cup butter
- 2 tbsp minced garlic
- A pinch of red pepper flakes
- 1 tsp basil leaf (dried)

Instructions:

1. Preheat oven to 375 degrees F
2. Lay Foil Sheet. Place each filet of fish over one foil sheet,
3. Put your salmon on the foil
4. In a bowl, mix butter, basil, red pepper and garlic
5. Microwave 1 minute until butter is melted, stir well
6. Spread butter mixture evenly over the fish
7. Squeeze lemon over each filet
8. Wrap in foil, place on baking sheet
9. Bake for 15-17 minutes, until desired doneness is reached
10. Flip side to broil on high
11. Broil 1-2 minutes to crisp up edges of salmon
12. Serve it!
13. Cheers!

Nutrition Facts (Per serving):

•	**Calories**	513
•	**Sodium**	263mg
•	**Fat**	36.9g
•	**Potassium**	919mg
•	**Carbohydrate**	4.1g
•	**Fiber**	0.9g
•	**Sugars**	0.8g
•	**Protein**	44g
•	**Cholesterol**	159mg
•	**Calcium**	101mg
•	**Iron**	2mg

Blueberry Salmon Salad

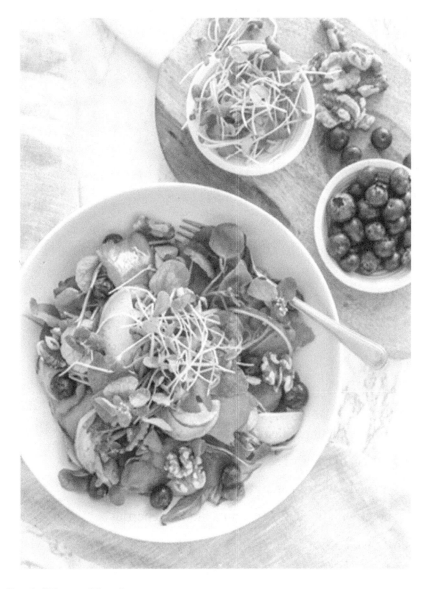

Prep Time: 15 min   Cook Time: 15 min

Servings: 4

Ingredients:

- 170g smoked salmon
- 2 ½ cups baby spinach – wash and trim
- 2 cups watercress
- ¼ cup raw unsalted walnut halves

- ½ cup fresh blueberries
- 1/2 small avocado (sliced/diced)
- 3 tbsp thinly sliced red onion
- Garnish: sprouts-radish, pea, sunflower
- Ginger citrus
- 1/2 cup extra virgin olive oil
- 1/3 cup freshly-squeezed orange juice
- 1 tbsp thinly sliced fresh mint and basil
- 2 tbsp apple cider vinegar
- 2 tsp mustard
- 1 tsp fresh ginger - finely grated
- 2 tsp raw honey
- black pepper to taste
- Sea salt to taste

Instructions:

1. Make the dressing: Mix all the ingredients in a small container
2. Add black pepper and few pinches of sea salt to taste. Set aside
3. Pat-dry the greens (spinach) with a paper towel
4. Place them in a big bowl with the herbs (walnuts and blueberries)
5. Add the dressing. Mix well
6. Add avocado, then divide the greens into two bowls
7. Arrange the smoked salmon pieces in the bowls. Garnish with the sprouts
8. Serve it!
9. Cheers!

Nutrition Facts (Per serving):

• **Calories**	429
• **Sodium**	1060mg

•	**Fat**	35.4g
•	**Potassium**	290mg
•	**Carbohydrate**	20.6g
•	**Fiber**	6.4g
•	**Sugars**	8.3g
•	**Protein**	11.8g
•	**Cholesterol**	10mg
•	**Calcium**	72mg
•	**Iron**	4mg

Turmeric falafel

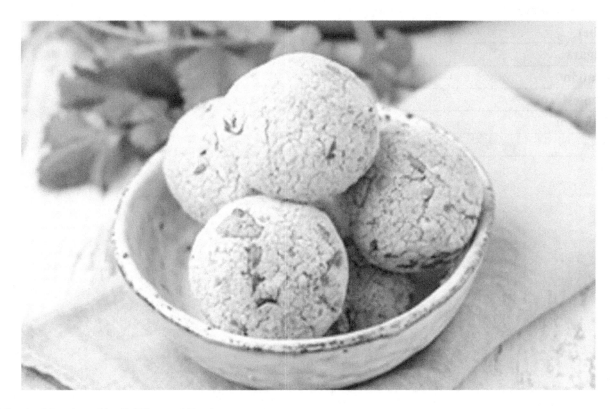

Prep Time: 10 min   Cook Time: 35 min

Servings: 3 (2 medium-size balls per serving)

Ingredients:

- 1 14-can chickpeas
- 2 tbsp Aquafaba (liquid from a can of chickpeas)
- 1 handful fresh cilantro or parsley
- 1 garlic clove
- 1 tsp turmeric
- 1 tsp olive oil
- Salt and pepper – to taste

Instructions:

1. Preheat oven to 390 degrees F

2. Combine all ingredients in a blender or food processor

3. Blend until smooth

4. Form balls with your hands

5. Bake for 20 minutes

6. Serve it!

7. Cheers!

Nutrition Facts (Per serving):

• **Calories**	497
• **Sodium**	869mg
• **Fat**	8.3g
• **Potassium**	1300mg
• **Carbohydrate**	83g
• **Fiber**	24g
• **Sugars**	14.5g
• **Protein**	26.4g
• **Cholesterol**	0mg
• **Calcium**	171mg
• **Iron**	10mg

Green edamame spinach hummus pesto

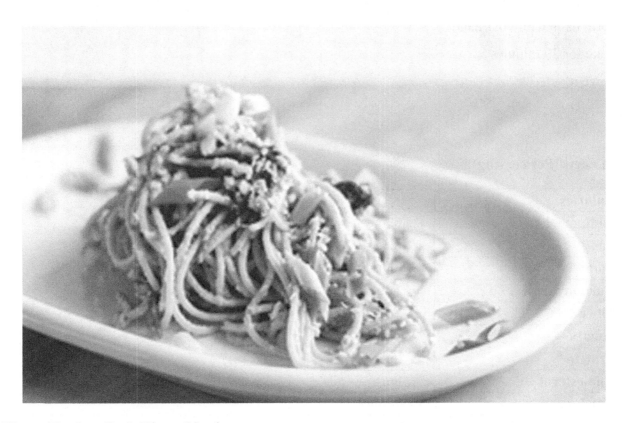

Prep Time: 10 min   Cook Time: 20 min

Serving: 2

Ingredients:

- 1 ¾ cups cooked edamame beans
- 7 ounces fresh spinach
- 1 tbsp tahini
- 1 tbsp lemon juice
- 2-3 garlic cloves, roughly chopped
- 2 spring onions, roughly chopped
- 2 tbsp nutritional yeast
- 1 tsp dried oregano
- Salt and pepper – to taste

Instructions:

1. Mix all the ingredients, except the spinach, in a blender or food processor until smooth.

2. Without oil, sauté the spinach on medium-high heat until wilted

3. Add a bit of water if needed

4. Fold in the spinach in the edamame mix and serve over pasta

5. Cheers!

Nutrition Facts (Per serving):

• **Calories**	178
• **Sodium**	235mg
• **Fat**	7g
• **Potassium**	900mg
• **Carbohydrate**	17.5g
• **Fiber**	8.1g
• **Sugars**	1.6g
• **Protein**	13.1g
• **Cholesterol**	0mg
• **Calcium**	204mg
• **Iron**	6mg

Deep dish falafel pizza

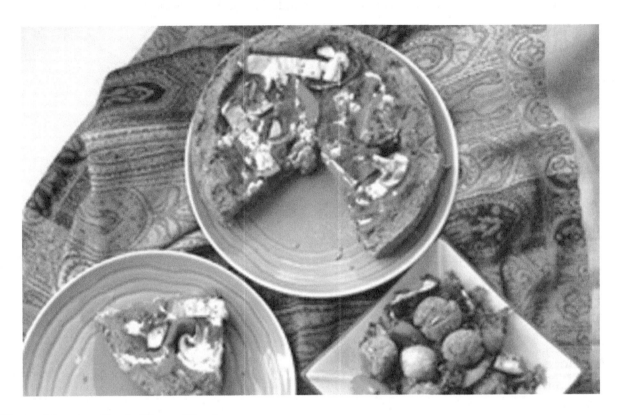

Prep Time: 20 min   Cook Time: 90 min

Servings: 4 (2 slices per serving)

Ingredients for the falafel:

- ¾ cup cooked chickpeas
- 1/3 cup millet, oats or flour
- 1 cup fresh coriander
- 1 cup fresh mint
- 1 small red onion
- 2 cloves garlic
- 3 tbsp tahini
- 3 tbsp ground chia or flex seeds
- 2 tbsp cumin
- 2 tbsp coriander powder

Ingredients for the beet hummus:

- ½ cup cooked chickpeas
- 2 tbsp tahini
- 1 clove garlic
- 1 small beet, boiled
- Oregano, basil and other herbs, as desired
- Sliced vegetables, as desired

Ingredients for the tahini cheese sauce:

- 2 tbsp tahini
- Nutritional yeast – to taste

Instructions:

1. Preheat oven to 390 degrees F

To make the base

2. Line a pie dish or cake pan with baking paper
3. In a food processor, pulse all crust ingredients to little pieces and well combined
4. Spread evenly over pie dish/cake pan
5. Bake in oven for 20 minutes

To make beet hummus

6. Pulse all the ingredients in food processor until smooth
7. Remove the beet hummus. Mix well with the sliced vegetables
8. Remove the falafel crust from oven when is dry to the touch,
9. Spread the beet hummus even over the crust.
10. Cook in oven for 40 minutes

To make the cheese sauce

11. Mix all ingredients and drizzle on top of pizza after baking.
12. Slice and serve
13. Cheers!

Nutrition Facts (Per serving):

• Calories	462
• Sodium	83mg
• Fat	16.6g
• Potassium	1085mg
• Carbohydrate	63.9g
• Fiber	21g
• Sugars	10.5g
• Protein	24.6g
• Cholesterol	0mg
• Calcium	312mg
• Iron	12mg

Crunchy fresh broccoli quinoa salad

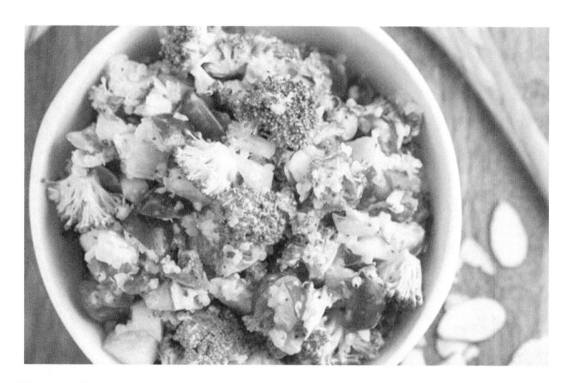

Prep Time: 20 min   Cook Time: 15 min

Servings: 4

Ingredients:

- 1 cucumber, seeded and diced (about 1 ¾ cups)
- 2 cups kale, white parts removed and chopped
- ½ small red onion, finely diced
- 2 cups seedless red grapes, cut into four
- 1 head broccoli, cut into small florets (2 cups)
- ½ cup slivered almonds
- 1 cup cooked quinoa ($^{1}/_{3}$ cup dry), cooled
- ¼ tsp freshly ground black pepper
- 2 tsp apple cider vinegar
- 1 tsp poppy seeds
- 2 tbsp vegan mayonnaise

- ½ tsp ground sea salt

- 1 tbsp agave nectar

- 1 ½ tbsp lemon juice

Instructions:

1. Prepare and chop ingredients

2. Add broccoli, cucumber, almonds, kale, red onion, grapes and quinoa to a large bowl

3. In a small container, mix apple cider vinegar, lemon juice, mayonnaise, agave, poppy seeds, salt and pepper. Stir with a spoon and add the dressing to the vegetable. Mix well

4. Serve it!

5. Cheers!

Nutrition Facts (Per serving):

• **Calories**	354
• **Sodium**	132mg
• **Fat**	10.9g
• **Potassium**	926mg
• **Carbohydrate**	56.1g
• **Fiber**	7.4g
• **Sugars**	16.3g
• **Protein**	12.1g
• **Cholesterol**	0mg
• **Calcium**	152mg
• **Iron**	4mg

Kale and chickpea stuffed spaghetti squash

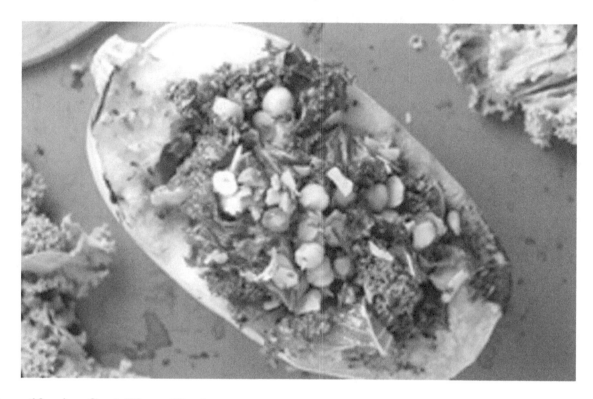

Prep Time: 10 min   Cook Time: 50 min

Servings: 3

Ingredients:

- 1 spaghetti squash
- 4-5 handfuls of kale, washed and large stems removed
- 2 cloves of garlic, minced
- 1 cup of chickpeas - drained and rinsed
- ¼ cup of almonds
- 1 tbsp Extra virgin olive oil
- Sea salt and pepper to taste

Instructions:

1. Preheat your oven to 390 degrees F

2. Cut spaghetti squash into half. Scoop out the seeds and strings

3. Coat the inside of the squash halves with olive oil. Sprinkle with sea salt and pepper

4. Place the squash halves facing down on a baking sheet – bake for 40 minutes

5. Meanwhile, drizzle olive oil into a pan over medium heat

6. Add the minced garlic and saute until the garlic turn golden.

7. Add the almonds and saute for another 3 minutes - until the almonds are just starting to toast

8. Add the kale. Sprinkle a little sea salt and saute until wilted,

9. Add the almonds and chickpeas. Mix well

10. Portion the kale mixture into the squash halves

11. Serve it!

12. Cheers!

Nutrition Facts (Per serving):

• Calories	376
• Sodium	41mg
• Fat	12.6g
• Potassium	979mg
• Carbohydrate	52.4g
• Fiber	15.2g
• Sugars	7.8g
• Protein	17.3g
• Cholesterol	0mg
• Calcium	167mg
• Iron	6mg

Beet and Quinoa Burgers

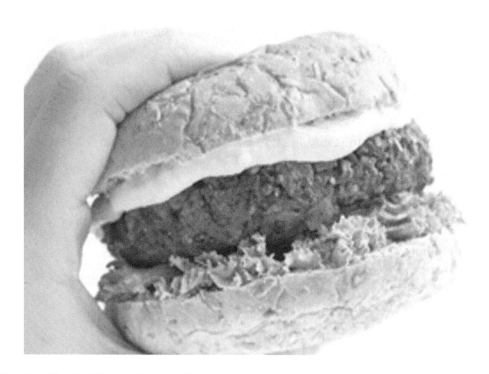

Prep Time: 15 min   Cook Time: 1 hour 45 min

Serving: 8

Ingredients:

- 1 ½ cups chopped eggplant
- 5 tbsp flax meal - divided
- 6 tbsp warm water
- 1 cup cooked quinoa
- 4 cups shredded beets
- 1 cup gluten-free rolled oats
- ½ cup hummus
- 2 garlic cloves, minced
- Salt and pepper – to taste
- 1 tbsp Cooking oil

Instructions:

1. Put the eggplant into a steaming basket and steam until tender - about 5 minutes. Transfer to a food processor and process until smooth. Transfer to a mixing bowl and set aside.

2. In a small bowl, add 2 tbsps of flax meal and water. Mix well and set aside.

3. Add remaining 3 tbsp of flax meal, beets, oats, quinoa, and garlic into a large mixing bowl. Mix Well. Pour the mixture into a food processor to process. Transfer back to the bowl.

4. Add the water, eggplant and hummus into the bowl. Mix until it forms dough - you can shape it into patties. Add salt and pepper. If it seems too wet, add more flax to let the oats and flax soak up some of the liquid.

5. Line a baking sheet with parchment paper and divide the dough into 8 patties. Put in refrigerator and let chill for at least 60 minutes.

6. To cook the burgers, heat up a little oil in a large skillet over medium heat. Sear the burgers until brown, about 3-4 minutes. Repeat until all burgers are done.

7. Top with greens and a smear of hummus.

8. Serve with your gluten-free buns.

9. Cheers!

Nutrition Facts (Per serving):

• **Calories**	203
• **Sodium**	127mg
• **Fat**	6.7g
• **Potassium**	468mg
• **Carbohydrate**	0mg
• **Fiber**	6.6g
• **Sugars**	7.2g
• **Protein**	7.7g
• **Cholesterol**	0mg
• **Calcium**	41mg
• **Iron**	3mg

Sweet potato "rice" in Deep Dish

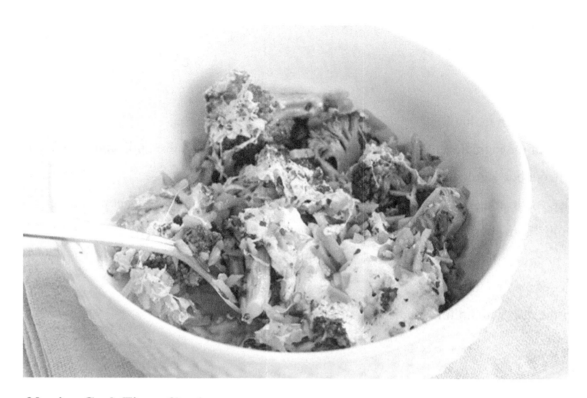

Prep Time: 20 min   Cook Time: 60 min

Servings: 4

Ingredients:

Pesto

- 2 ½ cups basil leaves
- 3 tbsp pine nuts
- ¼ cup olive oil
- 5 cranks of a sea salt grinder
- 5 cranks of peppercorn grinder
- 1 large garlic clove, minced

For the rest

- 2 cups small broccoli florets
- 1 large sweet potato, peeled and spiralized

- Pepper – to taste
- $^1/_3$ cup low-sodium vegetable broth
- 1 ½ cups shredded vegan mozzarella

Instructions:

1. Preheat the oven to 400 F
2. Place all of the ingredients for the pesto into a food processor and pulse until smooth. Pour 1/2 of the pesto into a bowl. Add in the broccoli. Mix well. Set aside.
3. In a deep dish, spread out a thin layer of pesto followed by a layer of the sweet potato rice. Then, add the broccoli. Then, cover broccoli with the rest of the rice. Put the remaining pesto evenly over the rice. Then, pour over the vegetable broth. Season with pepper. If using mozzarella, spread over in an even layer over the rice to covert.
4. Cover the dish with tin foil and bake for 40 minutes
5. Serve it!
6. Cheers!

Nutrition Facts (Per serving):

• Calories	301
• Sodium	285mg
• Fat	7.7g
• Potassium	268mg
• Carbohydrate	6g
• Fiber	1.7g
• Sugars	1.5g
• Protein	12.2g
• Cholesterol	33mg
• Calcium	265mg
• Iron	1mg

Golden roasted cauliflower and chickpeas

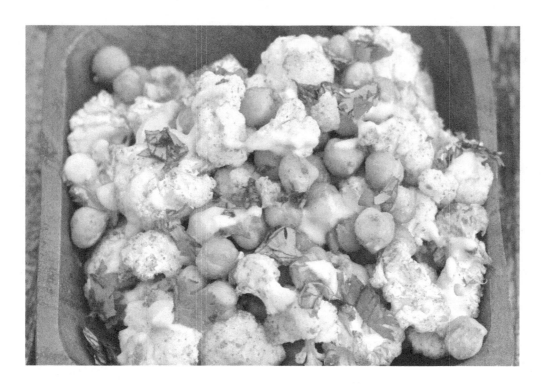

Prep Time: 15 min   Cook Time: 40 min

Servings: 3

Ingredients:

- 1 head cauliflower, cut into florets
- 1 ½ cups cooked chickpeas
- 2 tbsp olive oil
- 2 garlic cloves, minced
- 1 ½ tsp ground turmeric
- 1 tsp ground cumin
- 1 tsp ground coriander
- ½ tsp salt
- ¼ cup chopped fresh cilantro for garnish, if desired
- Lemon-tahini dressing, optional

Instructions:

1. Preheat oven to 400 degrees F
2. Toss all ingredients together in a large bowl until cauliflower and chickpeas are evenly coated
3. Spread onto a large baking sheet lined with foil and roast about 25 minutes, until tender
4. Serve as a side dish or over a warm bed of quinoa as a main dish
5. Cheers!

Nutrition Facts (Per serving):

• **Calories**	476
• **Sodium**	440mg
• **Fat**	15.7g
• **Potassium**	1192mg
• **Carbohydrate**	67g
• **Fiber**	20g
• **Sugars**	12.9g
• **Protein**	21.4g
• **Cholesterol**	0mg
• **Calcium**	137mg
• **Iron**	8mg

Curried Tofu

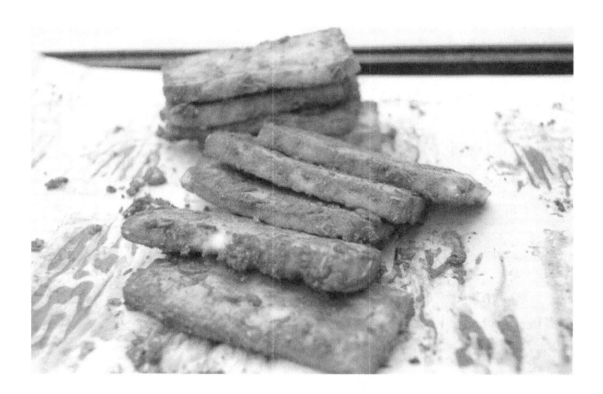

Prep Time: 10 min   Cook Time: 1 hour 35 min

Servings: 2 (4 pieces per serving)

Ingredients:

For the tofu

- 1 block firm tofu

For the marinade

- 2 tbsp soy sauce
- 3 tbsp water
- ½ tsp garam masala
- ½ tsp turmeric powder
- ½ tsp curry powder
- ½ tsp onion powder

- ½ tsp cumin seeds
- 2 garlic cloves, grated

Instructions:

1. Add all the marinade ingredients to a mixing bowl and mix with a whisk. Set aside.
2. Cut the tofu into strips, place them in the marinade. Leaves for 30 minutes.
3. Preheat the oven to 350°F.
4. Place the tofu strips in a single row on a parchment covered baking sheet.
5. Bake for 25 minutes. Flip side. Bake for an additional 20 minutes
6. Server it!
7. Cheers!

Nutrition Facts (Per serving):

• Calories	52
• Sodium	911mg
• Fat	2.2g
• Potassium	151mg
• Carbohydrate	4.3g
• Fiber	1g
• Sugars	0.8g
• Protein	5.2g
• Cholesterol	0mg
• Calcium	111mg
• Iron	2mg

Anti-inflammatory Snacks

Coconut and sweet potato muffins with cinnamon, ginger and maple syrup

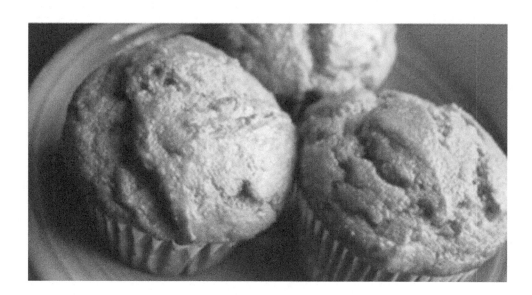

Prep Time: 20 min   Cook Time: 1 hour 50 min

Servings: 8 medium cups

Ingredients:

- 1 small organic sweet potato, roasted (1 cup, packed)
- 3 organic free-range eggs, lightly beaten
- ¾ cup of organic canned coconut milk
- ¼ cup of organic coconut flour
- 1 cup of organic brown rice flour
- ½ cup of pure organic maple syrup
- 1 tbsp baking powder
- ½ tsp pink Himalayan salt
- 1 tbsp of ground cinnamon
- ⅛ tsp of ground cloves

- ⅛ tsp of ground nutmeg

- 1 tsp of ground ginger

- 2 tbsp of organic olive oil

Instructions:

1. Preheat oven to 400 degrees F.

2. Oil a muffin tray.

3. Poke holes in your sweet potato and place in oven – cook for 60 minutes (or until soft).

4. Remove sweet potato from oven. Let cool.

5. Peel the sweet potato and place the rest in a mixing bowl.

6. Add maple syrup, coconut milk, beaten eggs and olive oil to the sweet potato. Mix until smooth.

7. Mix the dry ingredients in a separate bowl.

8. Add the dry ingredients to the sweet potato. Mix well.

9. Pour the batter in the muffin pan and fill each hole until ⅔ full.

10. Cook in oven for 30 minutes.

11. To test if it's well done, insert knife in the middle of the muffin and it should come out clean.

12. Serve it!

13. Cheers!

Nutrition Facts (Per serving):

• **Calories**	259
• **Sodium**	71mg
• **Fat**	11.8g
• **Potassium**	418mg
• **Carbohydrate**	35.6g
• **Fiber**	3.8g
• **Sugars**	14.7g
• **Protein**	5.1g
• **Cholesterol**	70mg
• **Calcium**	106mg
• **Iron**	2mg

Golden milk chia pudding

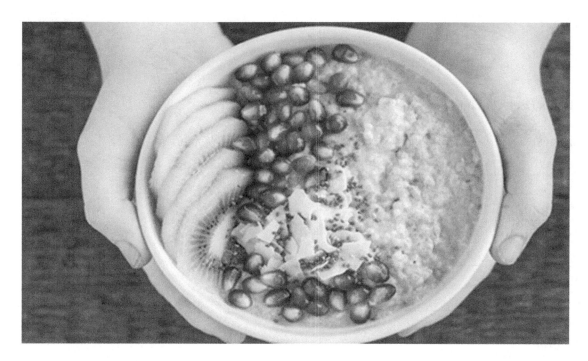

Prep Time: 10 min   Cook Time: 15 min

Servings: 4

Ingredients:

- 1 can full fat coconut milk
- 1/4 tsp cinnamon powder
- 1/4 tsp cardamom powder
- 1 1/4 tsp turmeric powder
- 1/4 tsp ginger powder
- 3 pinches of black pepper
- 1 tbsp maple syrup
- 6 tbsp of chia seeds

Instructions:

1. Put all ingredients (EXCEPT CHIA SEEDS) into blender. Process until creamy smooth.
2. Whisk in chia seeds and pour into glass jar.

3. Refrigerate overnight.

4. Top with favorite toppings.

5. Serve it!

6. Cheers!

Nutrition Facts (Per serving):

• **Calories**	91
• **Sodium**	8mg
• **Fat**	7.4g
• **Potassium**	56mg
• **Carbohydrate**	6.5g
• **Fiber**	1.5g
• **Sugars**	3.5g
• **Protein**	1.3g
• **Cholesterol**	0mg
• **Calcium**	36mg
• **Iron**	1mg

Golden turmeric milk chia seed pudding

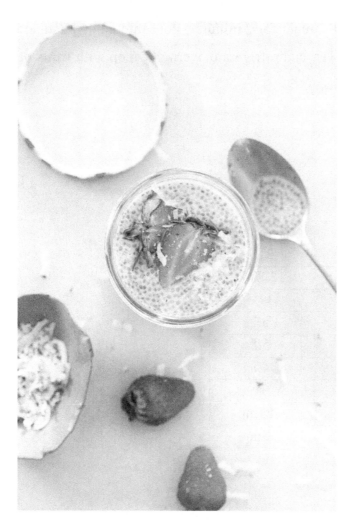

Prep Time: 10 min   Cook Time: 10 min

Servings: 4 cups

Ingredients:

- 2 cups Coconut Milk
- 1/2 tsp Cinnamon Powder
- 1/2 tsp Turmeric Powder
- 1/2 tbsp Maple Syrup
- 3 tbsp Chia Seeds

Instructions:

1. In a saucepan add coconut milk, cinnamon powder, turmeric powder and maple syrup

2. Bring to quick boil and simmer for 2 minutes. Pour into a bowl and add chia seeds. Mix well.

3. Pour into two separate jars and refrigerate overnight. Top with fruits of your choice. Serve cold in the morning for breakfast.

4. Cheers!

Nutrition Facts (Per serving):

• **Calories**	313
• **Sodium**	18mg
• **Fat**	31.2g
• **Potassium**	377mg
• **Carbohydrate**	11.5g
• **Fiber**	5.2g
• **Sugars**	5.5g
• **Protein**	4.3g
• **Cholesterol**	0mg
• **Calcium**	81mg
• **Iron**	3mg

Paleo ginger spiced muffins

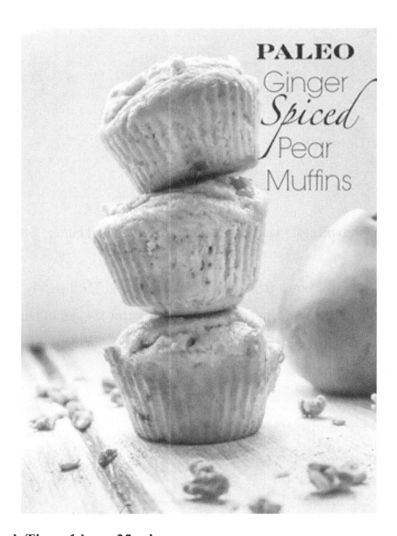

Prep Time: 15 min   Cook Time: 1 hour 35 min

Servings: 12 (small cup)

Ingredients:

- 3 small Pears
- 1 tbsp cinnamon
- 1 tbsp butter or melted coconut oil
- 1/4 cup and 1 tbsp honey (You'll use 1 tbsp separately)
- 1/4 cup natural Ginger-ale
- 1 tbsp ground ginger

- 1 1/2 cup almond meal
- 1/4 cup coconut flour
- 1/2 cup potato starch
- 1 tsp baking powder
- 3 eggs
- Sprinkle of sea salt
- 1/4 cup nuts or seeds (Optional)

Instructions:

1. Peel your pears. Chop into pieces. Place in bowl and mix in melted butter, 1 tbsp honey and ginger ale. Let that soak.
2. Put eggs and spices in another bowl. Beat until it become fluffy. Then slowly add in flours nuts, baking powder. Mix well. Add in pear and ginger mixture and an extra 1/4 cup of honey. Mix again.
3. Fill oiled muffins cups with batter. Bake in oven at 350F for 25 minutes -- until muffins turn golden brown. Let cool and top with more cinnamon.
4. Serve it!
5. Cheers!

Nutrition Facts (Per serving):

• **Calories**	195
• **Sodium**	28mg
• **Fat**	8.4g
• **Potassium**	200mg
• **Carbohydrate**	29g
• **Fiber**	4.4g
• **Sugars**	14.9g
• **Protein**	4.8g
• **Cholesterol**	43mg
• **Calcium**	67mg
• **Iron**	1mg

Winter fruit salad

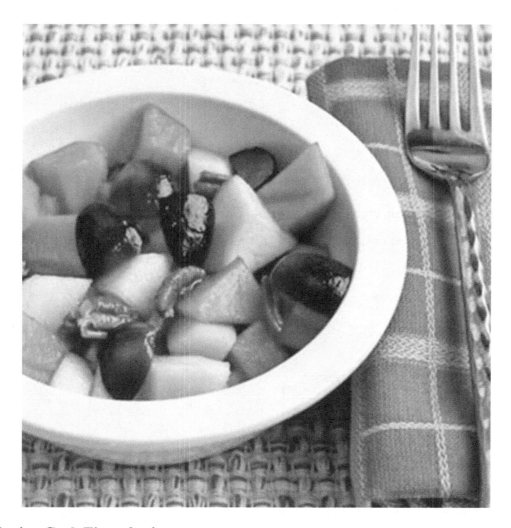

Prep Time: 25 min   Cook Time: 0 min

Servings: 6

Ingredients:

- 3 Bosch pears, cut into cubes (enough to make 2 cups)

- 4 persimmons, cut into cubes (enough to make 2 cups)

- 3/4 cup pecans, cut into half-length to make slivers

- 1 cup grapes, cut into halves (May replaced with other fruits such as apples, pomegranate or figs - 5-6 cups of cut fruit needed)

Dressing Ingredients:

- 1 tbsp peanut oil

- 1 tbsp extra virgin olive oil

- 2 tbsp agave nectar (you may use pomegranate molasses instead)

- 1 tbsp pomegranate-flavored red wine vinegar

- pinch of salt, to taste

Instructions:

1. Whisk together the dressing ingredients so flavors can blend while you cut the fruit.

2. Place cut grapes, persimmons, and pears in plastic bowl. Toss fruit with dressing. Toss with pecan pieces and serve.

3. Cheers!

Nutrition Facts (Per serving):

• **Calories**	171
• **Sodium**	2mg
• **Fat**	1.2g
• **Potassium**	192mg
• **Carbohydrate**	22.5g
• **Fiber**	3.2g
• **Sugars**	12g
• **Protein**	1.2g
• **Cholesterol**	0mg
• **Calcium**	18mg
• **Iron**	1mg

Coconut turmeric bites

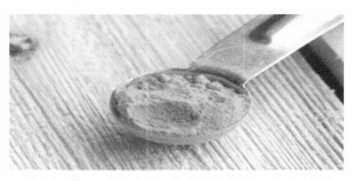

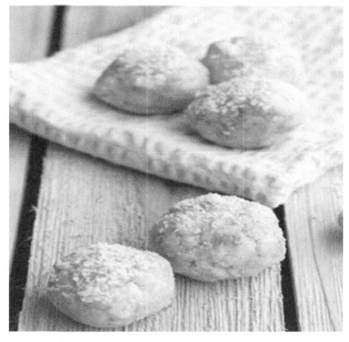

Prep Time: 15 min   Cook Time: 50 min

Servings: 6

Ingredients:

- 3/4 cup coconut butter (also called coconut cream concentrate or coconut mana)
- 3/4 cup shredded coconut + 1/2 tsp for topping (I highly recommend tropical traditions for this)
- 1 tbsp coconut milk (or water)
- 1 tsp coconut oil

- 2 tsp turmeric
- 1/2 tsp cinnamon
- Pinch of black pepper (omit for strict AIP)
- 1 tbsp honey (optional: it helps to balance the bitter taste of the turmeric)

Instructions:

1. In a mixing bowl, add the coconut butter and shredded coconut. Mix well. Coconut butter should be softened but not melted.
2. Add the remaining ingredients. Mix them to make dough.
3. Roll the dough into balls about 1 1/4″ in diameter. Place onto a plate lined with parchment paper. If desired, sprinkle 1/2 tsp of shredded coconut on top.
4. Put the turmeric bites into the refrigerator and chill for 30 minutes.
5. Remove from the fridge and serve!
6. Cheers!

Nutrition Facts (Per serving):

• **Calories**	271
• **Sodium**	14mg
• **Fat**	25g
• **Potassium**	87mg
• **Carbohydrate**	13.2g
• **Fiber**	6.8g
• **Sugars**	5.9g
• **Protein**	2.7g
• **Cholesterol**	0mg
• **Calcium**	14mg
• **Iron**	4mg

Strawberry chia seed jam

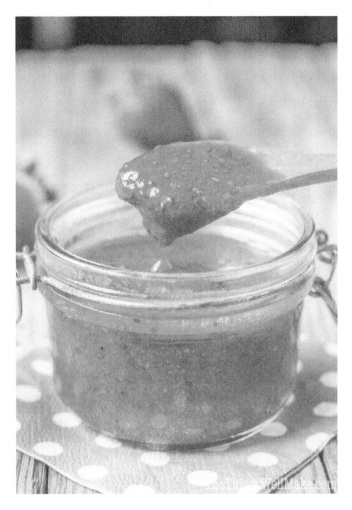

Prep Time: 10 min   Cook Time: 60 min

Servings: 20 (To apply on bread)

Ingredients:

- 2 cup strawberries - washed and chopped into smaller pieces
- 1/2 lime - juiced
- 2 tbsp chia seeds
- 1 tbsp vanilla extract
- 1 tbsp honey or maple syrup

Instructions:

1. Add the berries to a saucepan over medium heat. Cook until the berries are softened.

2. Add in the honey or syrup along with the lime juice. Stir over the stove until they are well combined. Press against them with a wooden spatula to help make more of a lumpy sauce.

3. Remove the pan from the heat. Add in the chia seeds and vanilla extract. Vanilla gave a depth of flavor that changed the jam for the better.

4. Stir in the chia seeds and wait a couple of minutes for it to become gel like. Add in more chia seeds, a little at a time, to make it looks thicker.

5. Store in the refrigerator for a week. The jam will slightly thicken up when cold.

6. Serve it!

7. Cheers!

Nutrition Facts (Per serving):

• Calories	16
• Sodium	0.3mg
• Fat	0.6g
• Potassium	35mg
• Carbohydrate	2.8g
• Fiber	0.8g
• Sugars	1.7g
• Protein	0.4g
• Cholesterol	0mg
• Calcium	15mg
• Iron	0.2mg

Smooth chocolate chia pudding

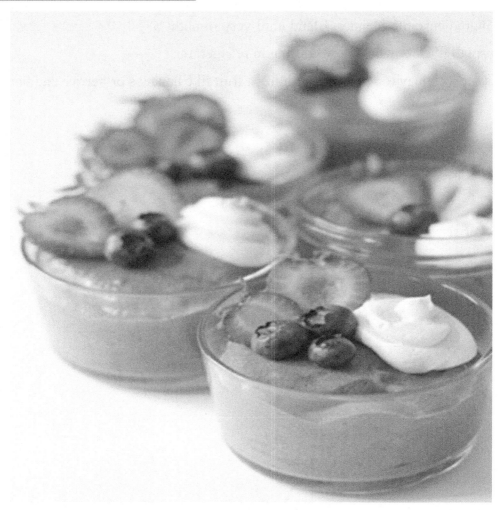

Prep Time: 15 min   Cook Time: 0 min

Servings: 6 (Medium-size cup)

Ingredients:

- 1 cup chia seeds
- 1/3 tsp ground cinnamon
- 2 1/4 cups glass-fed or organic milk (May use full-fat coconut milk)
- 1/3 cup cacao powder
- 1 tsp organic vanilla extract
- 1/4 cup honey
- 1/4 tsp sea salt

Instructions:

1. Place all ingredients into blender. Blend until very smooth

2. Pour into small glass bowls. Allow chilling in refrigerator

3. To add flavor, you may top pudding with fresh fruit like bananas or berries and homemade whipped cream

4. Serve it!

5. Cheers!

Nutrition Facts (Per serving):

• **Calories**	193
• **Sodium**	122mg
• **Fat**	10.5g
• **Potassium**	193mg
• **Carbohydrate**	29.3g
• **Fiber**	9.8g
• **Sugars**	15.8g
• **Protein**	9.1g
• **Cholesterol**	8mg
• **Calcium**	281mg
• **Iron**	3mg

Pomegranate ginger gummies

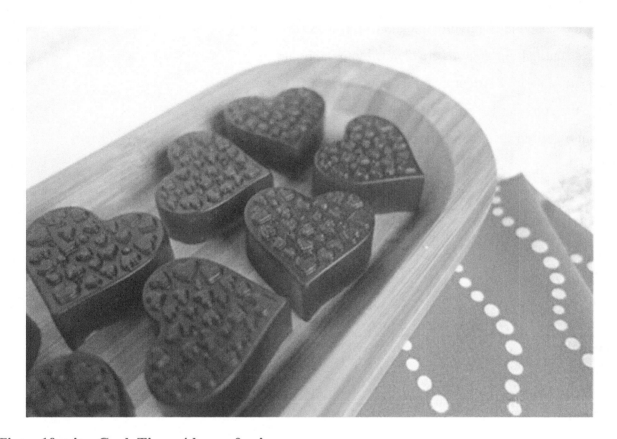

Prep Time: 10 min   Cook Time: 4 hours 0 min

Servings: 15 (small pieces)

Ingredients:

- 1/2 cup lemon juice
- 1 cup pomegranate juice
- 1/2 cup water
- 1 tbsp honey
- 1/2 inch ginger, grated
- 6 tbsp grass-fed gelatin

Instructions:

1. Place the pomegranate juice, lemon juice, ginger, honey and water in a large saucepan. Heat it to a simmer.

2. Pour the heated juice mixture into a blender. Add the gelatin.

3. Process until all the gelatins are blended into the liquid.

4. Pour into a mold. Refrigerate for 2 hours.

5. Once the gummies have firmed up, pop them out of the mold.

6. Cut into desired shapes and serve.

7. Cheers!

Nutrition Facts (Per serving):

• Calories	23
• Sodium	10mg
• Fat	0.1
• Potassium	33mg
• Carbohydrate	3g
• Fiber	0.1g
• Sugars	2.6g
• Protein	2.6g
• Cholesterol	0mg
• Calcium	2mg
• Iron	0.3mg

Baked zucchini chips

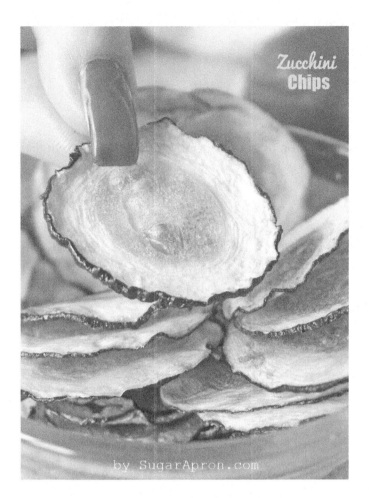

Prep Time: 15 min   Cook Time: 1 hour 30 min

Servings: 2 (7-8 slices per serving)

Ingredients:

- 1 large zucchini
- 2 tbsp olive oil
- Salt – to taste

Instructions:

1. Preheat oven to 225 degrees F. Line two large baking sheets with parchment paper. Set aside.

2. Slice zucchini in the thickness of a quarter (to about 15 slices)

3. Sandwich the zucchini slices between 2 paper towels and press on them. This helps draw out the liquid to speed up the cooking time.

4. Lay out slices on prepared baking sheet, tightly next to each other in a straight line. Ensure no overlapping.

5. Brush the olive oil on each zucchini slice.

6. Sprinkle with salt.

7. Bake in oven for 45 minutes. Flip over slices. Bake for another 45 minutes, until they start to turn brown.

8. Let cool before serving.

9. Cheers!

Nutrition Facts (Per serving):

• **Calories**	146
• **Sodium**	94mg
• **Fat**	14.3
• **Potassium**	423mg
• **Carbohydrate**	5.4g
• **Fiber**	1.8g
• **Sugars**	2.8g
• **Protein**	2g
• **Cholesterol**	0mg
• **Calcium**	24mg
• **Iron**	1mg

Anti-inflammatory Smoothies

Cherry Mango Smoothie

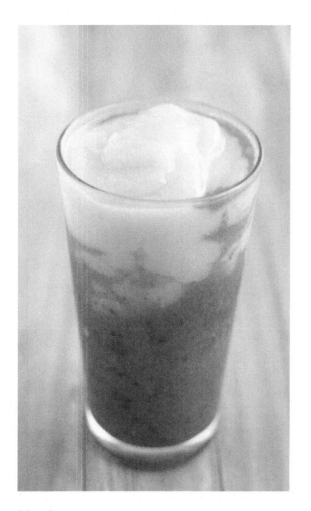

Prep Time: 5 min   Cook Time: 10 min

Servings: 2

Ingredients:

- 1 cup frozen sweet cherries
- 1 1/2 cup water
- 1 cup frozen mango

Instructions:

1. Blend the cherries first: place the cherries and 1/2 cup water in the blender. Blend until smooth. Add another 1/4 cup water if it seems too thick.
2. Pour into a glass.
3. Repeat Step 1 for mango.
4. Pour into the glass on top of the cherry layer.
5. Serve it!
6. Cheers!

Nutrition Facts (Per serving):

• **Calories**	145
• **Sodium**	5mg
• **Fat**	0.7g
• **Potassium**	459mg
• **Carbohydrate**	36.6g
• **Fiber**	4.8g
• **Sugars**	27.3g
• **Protein**	2.1g
• **Cholesterol**	0mg
• **Calcium**	31mg
• **Iron**	0.4mg

Green smoothie

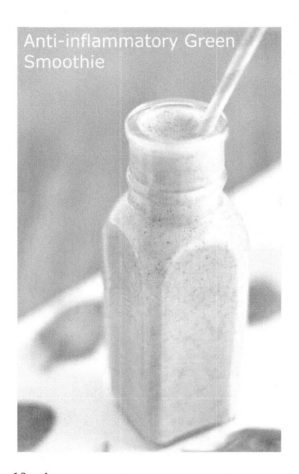

Prep Time: 5 min   Cook Time: 10 min

Servings: 2

Ingredients:

- 1 1/2 cup unsweetened almond milk
- 2 cups fresh spinach
- 1 slices frozen banana cut into small pieces
- 1/2 inch piece of fresh ginger - peeled and sliced
- 1/2 piece of fresh turmeric - peeled and sliced
- 1/2 tsp ground cinnamon
- 1 tsp flax seeds
- 1 tsp chia seeds

Instructions:

1. Place all ingredients in blender, Blend until smooth.

2. Pour into a glass and serve.

3. Cheers!

Nutrition Facts (Per serving):

• **Calories**	137
• **Sodium**	160mg
• **Fat**	5.7g
• **Potassium**	560mg
• **Carbohydrate**	21.3g
• **Fiber**	6.8g
• **Sugars**	7.5g
• **Protein**	4.1g
• **Cholesterol**	0mg
• **Calcium**	316mg
• **Iron**	3mg

Pineapple ginger turmeric smoothie

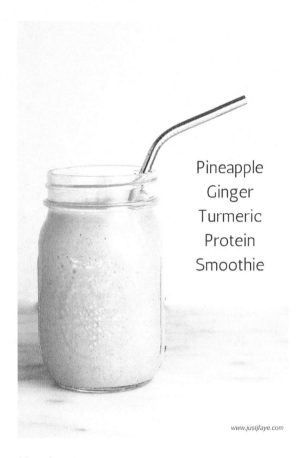

Pineapple
Ginger
Turmeric
Protein
Smoothie

www.justjfaye.com

Prep Time: 5 min   Cook Time: 10 min

Servings: 2

Ingredients:

- 1 cup frozen pineapple chunks
- ½ frozen banana
- 1 cup unsweetened almond milk
- 1 tbsp chia seeds
- ½ tsp fresh grated ginger
- ½ tsp turmeric
- 1 scoop protein powder

Instructions:

1. Add all the ingredients to a blender, blend until smooth
2. Cheers!

Nutrition Facts (Per serving):

• **Calories**	245
• **Sodium**	121mg
• **Fat**	4.5g
• **Potassium**	461mg
• **Carbohydrate**	40g
• **Fiber**	5.3g
• **Sugars**	30g
• **Protein**	14g
• **Cholesterol**	32mg
• **Calcium**	254mg
• **Iron**	2mg

Turmeric golden milk smoothie

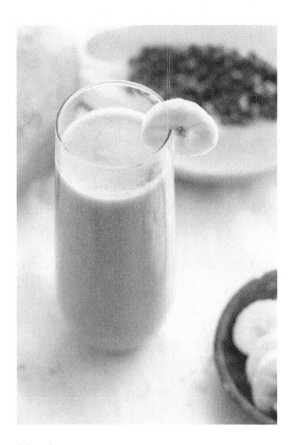

Prep Time: 10 min   Cook Time: 30 min

Servings: 2

Ingredients:

- 2 Cups Coconut or Almond Milk (plain)
- 1 tsp ground Turmeric
- Pinch of black pepper
- 1/2 tsp ground ginger
- 1 tbsp agave or maple syrup or honey

For smoothie

- brewed golden milk
- 1 banana (fresh or frozen)

- 1 cup frozen mango

- Half of a papaya (about 2 cups. Fresh or Frozen).

- 2 tbsp coconut cream (optional)

- vanilla (1 tsp or less)

Instructions:

1. First brew the golden milk.

2. Combine all your ingredients (the first 5 from the golden milk list) in a small saucepan. Bring to a quick boil and then reduce to low and simmer for 5 minutes. Whisk all together until blended.

3. Remove and let cool.

4. Combine your golden milk with the rest of you smoothie ingredients listed.

5. Blend fruit, coconut milk, golden milk, vanilla, etc.

6. Blend until smooth.

7. You may use pineapple in replacement for papaya.

8. Serve it!

9. Cheers!

Nutrition Facts (Per serving):

• **Calories**	315
• **Sodium**	17mg
• **Fat**	26.9g
• **Potassium**	340mg
• **Carbohydrate**	19.9g
• **Fiber**	7.5g
• **Sugars**	11g
• **Protein**	2.9g
• **Cholesterol**	0mg
• **Calcium**	11mg
• **Iron**	12mg

Kiwi smoothie

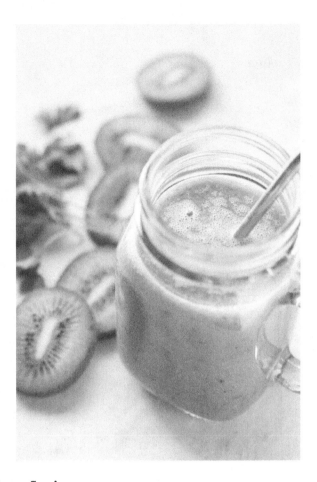

Prep Time: 10 min   Cook Time: 5 min

Servings: 2

Ingredients:

- 2 kiwis (peeled)
- 1 lemon (juiced)
- 1 lime (juiced)
- 4 oz orange juice
- 1 cup coconut water
- ice
- 1 sprig of parsley
- small handful of baby spinach - steam beforehand
- 1/2 tsp ground ginger

- 1 tbsp chia seed

- pinch of sea salt

- 1 tsp maple syrup or honey (optional)

Instructions:

1. Blend and add ice to serve.

2. Cheers!

Nutrition Facts (Per serving):

• **Calories**	196
• **Sodium**	277mg
• **Fat**	2.2g
• **Potassium**	762mg
• **Carbohydrate**	44.7g
• **Fiber**	8.4g
• **Sugars**	26.7g
• **Protein**	4.2g
• **Cholesterol**	0mg
• **Calcium**	131mg
• **Iron**	4mg

Frozen cranberry orange smoothie

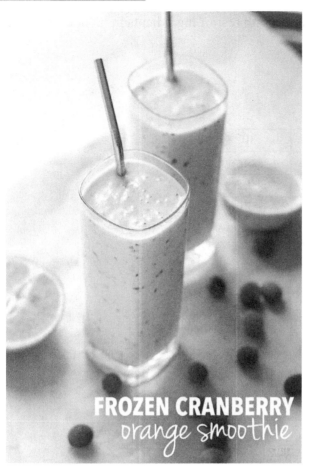

Prep Time: 5 min   Cook Time: 10 min

Servings: 3

Ingredients:

- 2 oz. fresh squeezed orange juice
- 1 small banana
- 2 cup frozen raw cranberries
- 1 tbsp lemon juice or few drops lemon essential oils
- 1 cup coconut or almond milk
- 1 tsp honey or maple syrup
- Optional - ice for more thickness or protein powder of choice.

Instructions:

1. Make orange juice. Put together with rest of ingredients in blender. Blend until smooth and serve.

2. Cheers!

Nutrition Facts (Per serving):

• **Calories**	302
• **Sodium**	13mg
• **Fat**	19.2g
• **Potassium**	657mg
• **Carbohydrate**	33g
• **Fiber**	4.1g
• **Sugars**	25.6g
• **Protein**	2.9g
• **Cholesterol**	0mg
• **Calcium**	28mg
• **Iron**	1mg

Conclusion

We have to remember the fact that we are what we eat. Researchers show that our health is dependent a lot on the food we eat; Of course not forgetting that we also need to work out to build up our muscles. Muscles are what you need to move your body.

Poor nutrition choices and hidden food allergies can cause inflammation in our bodies and can lead to a number of serious chronic diseases.

This book starts with explaining about inflammation, the different types of inflammatory diseases and the causes of the diseases. Follow on is a series of simple and tasty recipes that you can follow for your daily cooking.

We have to stay informed about the fact that we should limit processed foods, use spices and herbs in our diets instead of salt, eat whole grains instead of refined grains; and eat plenty of fresh fruits and vegetables; at least five times a day.

It's time to take action now. You are the only one that can make a change in your life.

Hurry! Purchase the ingredients listed in the recipes, get yourself in an apron and start preparing those delicious and healthy food. You and your love one deserves it!

Eat healthy every day and you will feel the difference in your life.

I hope that this guide is helpful to you!

Cheers!

-- [Melanie Finley]

Check Out Related Books

Go here to check out other related books that might interest you:

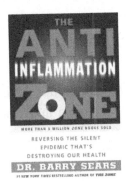

The Anti-Inflammation Zone

http://www.amazon.com/dp/B000FC2P6A

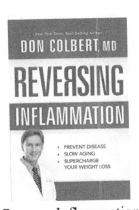

Reverse Inflammation

http://www.amazon.com/dp/B00Q1UF9UO

Made in the USA
Middletown, DE
22 August 2023

37140339R00060